CROSS TR

Father,

Thank you for the abilities you give us, for the strength and wisdom we gain from training.

Be with us as we work that we may do our best. Help us to be encouraging to others in our daily life. Thank you for the people that you have brought into our lives.

Bless the athletes, coaches, workout partners and all those who support our training.
May the results from our training be a reflection of Your Spirit in our lives.

Finally Father, remind us that there is no failure, but only growth in the body, mind and Spirit.

Amen

Contents

Copyright 4

Disclaimer 5

Bonus Content 6

Introduction 7

Benefits of Cross Training 8

Terminology 10

Beginner WODs 16

Benchmark – The Girls 23

Benchmark - Hero WODs 28

Bodyweight WODs 43

Running WODs 74

C2 Rowing WODs 79

Kettlebell WODs 83

Olympic Lifting WODs 96

Strongman WODs 102

Short 'N' Heavy WODs 107

Minute by Minute WODs 117

Bi-Element WODs 122

Tri-Element WODs 128

Four or More WODs 134

Hybrid WODs 140

AMRAP WODs 146

Epic Endurance Challenges 152

Conclusion 157

Copyright

Cross Training WOD Bible: 555 Workouts from Beginner to Ballistic

First Edition – March 2014.

Written by P Selter

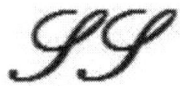

A Shredded-Society Publication
www.Shredded-Society.com
Copyright © 2014
All rights reserved.
This book or any portion thereof may not be reproduced or used in any manner whatsoever without the expressed written permission of the publisher except for the use of brief quotation in a book review.

Disclaimer

The information provided in this book is designed to provide helpful information on the subjects discussed. This book is not meant to be used, nor should it be used, to diagnose or treat any medical condition. For diagnosis or treatment of any medical problem, consult your own physician. The publisher and author are not responsible for any specific health or allergy needs that may require medical supervision and are not liable for any damages or negative consequences from any treatment, action, application or preparation, to any person reading or following the information in this book. References are provided for informational purposes only and do not constitute endorsement of any websites or other sources. Readers should be aware that the websites listed in this book may change.

I recommend consulting a doctor to assess and/or identify any health related issues prior to making any dramatic changes to your diet or exercise regime.

Bonus Content

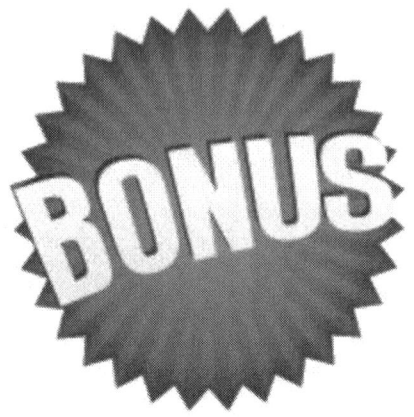

As a token of our appreciation Shredded-Society would like to give you access to our Cross Training exclusive bonus content.

You're only a click away from receiving:

The 5 most effective Cross Training workouts

A guide detailing the only Cross Training equipment you should use while training

Exclusive pre-release access to our latest eBooks

Free Shredded Society eBooks during promotional periods

Simply navigate to:

http://shredded-society.com/WOD.html

As this is a limited time offer it would be a shame to miss out, I recommend grabbing these bonuses before reading on.

Introduction

I would like to thank you and congratulate you for purchasing the book, Cross Training WOD Bible.

This book will introduce you to the many health & fitness benefits of the phenomenon that is Cross Training, along with 555 Cross Training WODs (workouts) you can implement immediately to improve your speed, strength and agility.

These workouts have been broken down into categories based on the content of each workout, these workouts range from beginner workouts that can be performed in the comfort of your own home or backyard to epic endurance challenges that will send you to the brink of both mental anguish and physical fatigue.

Thanks again for purchasing this book, I hope you enjoy it!

Benefits of Cross Training

Cross Training is not just a new fad amongst all the other styles of training that come and go throughout the years; Cross Training has many benefits these include:

Intensity

Cross Training workouts are fast paced and intense (as the emphasis is on speed and total weight being lifted), they are generally much shorter than a regular weight lifting workout – however since the workout is condensed it is constant non-stop movement, there is no time to stop and talk to your gym partner between sets like you normally would as you are constantly working against the clock to better yourself.

Creates Athletes

Cross Training exercises are all high power functional movements, this is highly emphasised. Cross Training, unlike bodybuilding does not believe in low power isolation movements. The major benefit here is now that the focus has been taken off vanity and looks it has been put 100% on performance – the core strength, stamina, coordination, agility and balance you will develop through participation in Cross Training will transfer over to sports and all other facets of life.

Time

The number one excuse for individuals not following a workout regime is the constraint of time; yes its true – working out takes time.
However, Cross Training WODs are short - with many intense workouts ranging from 15 – 20 minutes they are faster and

more effective than a regular workout in which you spend an hour on a cross trainer mindlessly staring at the wall.

Measureable Results

Cross Training workouts provide you with measureable and repeatable data; this can be used to verify that your fitness level is increasing. With a series of 'bench mark' workouts known as 'The Girls' and 'The Heroes' you can easily assess your progress.

Life Changing

Change your body, change your life, and change your world… Cross Training workouts build mental strength, grit and confidence; a tough Cross Training workout will emotionally push you beyond your limits. When you ignore the voice inside your head that says 'it's too hard' or 'I can't do that last rep' and push past it unbreakable confidence is built – then anything is possible.

Community

Cross Training encourages community, both in the gym and online.
People encourage and support each other through out their workouts – you will never have to work out alone again unless you want to, as the bond formed between training partners make training truly fun. It is very rarely you will find an individual that is as passionate about a particular pastime as yourself however this could not be further from the truth with the Cross Training community; we are all teammates that push and pray for each other.

Terminology

The following Cross Training terminology guide will come in helpful when interpreting your Cross Training workouts.

1RM: Your 1RM is your max lift for one rep

AHAP: as heavy as possible

AMRAP: As many rounds as possible

ATG: Ass to Grass

BP: Bench press

Box: Another name for a gym

BS: Back squat

BW: Body weight

CFT: Cross Training Total - consisting of max squat, press, and deadlift

CFWU: Cross Training Warm-up

Chipper: A WOD containing many different exercises and reps

CLN: Clean

C&J: Clean and jerk

C2: Concept II rowing machine

DL: Deadlift

DOMS: Delayed onset muscle soreness

DU: Double under

EMOM: Every minute on the minute

For Time: Timed workout, perform as quickly as possible and record score.

FS: Front squat

GHR(D): Glute ham raise (developer). Posterior chain exercise, similar to a back extension. Also, the device that allows for the proper performance of a Glute Ham Raise.

GHR(D) Situp: Situp performed on the GHR(D) bench.

GPP: General physical preparedness, another word for fitness

GTG: Grease the Groove, a protocol of doing many sub-maximal sets of an exercise throughout the day

H2H: Hand to hand; refers to Jeff Martone's kettlebell "juggling" techniques

HSPU: Hand stand push up. Kick up into a handstand (use wall for balance, if needed) bend arms until nose touches floor and push back up.

HSQ: Hang squat (clean or snatch). Start with bar "at the hang," about knee height. Initiate pull. As the bar rises drop into a full squat and catch the bar in the racked position. From there, rise to a standing position

IF: Intermittent Fasting

KB: Kettlebell

KBS: Kettlebell swing

KTE: Knees to elbows.

MetCon: Metabolic Conditioning workout

MP: Military press

MU: Muscle ups. Hanging from rings you do a combination pull-up and dip so you end in an upright support.

OH: Overhead

OHS: Overhead squat. Full-depth squat performed while arms are locked out in a wide grip press position above (and usually behind) the head.

PC: Power clean

Pd: Pood, weight measure for kettlebells

PR: Personal record

PP: Push press

PSN: Power snatch

PU: Pull-ups or push ups depending on the context in WOD

Rep: Repetition. One performance of an exercise.

RM: Repetition maximum.

ROM: Range of motion.

Rx'd: As prescribed, without any adjustments.

SDHP: Sumo deadlift high pull

Set: A number of repetitions. e.g., 34sets of 8 reps, often seen as 4x8, means you do 8 reps, rest, repeat, rest, repeat, rest, repeat.

SPP: Specific physical preparedness, aka skill training.

SN: Snatch

SQ: Squat

SS: Starting Strength; Mark Rippetoe's great book on strength training basics

Subbed: Substituted

T2B: Toes to bar. Hang from bar. Bending only at waist raise your toes to touch the bar, slowly lower them and repeat.

Tabata: A form of interval training comprised of 20 seconds on, 10 seconds off repeated for 8 rounds.

TGU: Turkish get-up

The Girls: A series of benchmark workouts named after girls

The Heroes: Brutal benchmark workouts in honour of fallen soldiers

TnG: Touch and go, no pausing between reps

WO: Workout

WOD: Workout of the day

YBF: You'll Be Fine

If a regular workout is a light cup of coffee that slowly wakes you up, Cross Training is a shot of five-hour energy!

Beginner WODs

The following 25 WODs require minimal equipment and are designed for newcomers to Cross Training & fitness in general.

Beginner Workout 1
3 rounds for time:
10 burpees
20 squats
30 situps

Beginner Workout 2
tabata (8 intervals – 20 seconds work – 10 seconds rest):
Pushups
Situps
Squats

Beginner Workout 3
5 rounds for time:
10 tuck jumps
15 back extensions

Beginner Workout 4
2 rounds for time:
400m run
50 lunges

Beginner Workout 5
For time:
100 pushups
50 situps

Beginner Workout 6
3 rounds for time:
20 burpees
30 squats
40 situps

Beginner Workout 7
4 rounds for time:
15 tuck jumps
25 situps

Beginner Workout 8
For time:
100 burpees

Beginner Workout 9
5 rounds for time:
20 burpees
10 situps
20 squats

Beginner Workout 10
For time:
5km run

Beginner Workout 11
For time:
50 box jumps
50 walking lunges
20 burpees

Beginner Workout 12
5 rounds for time:
20 jumping squats
20 sit ups
20 push ups

Beginner Workout 13
For time:
500m row
50 squats
40 sit ups
30 push ups
10 burpees

Beginner Workout 14
AMRAP
1 minute plank
15 bicycle crunches
10 burpees
1 minute plank
15 bicycle crunches
20 squats

Beginner Workout 15
3 rounds for time:
10 push ups
20 squats
10 crunches
10 burpees
25 jumping jacks
20 second plank
20 lunges

Beginner Workout 16
3 rounds for time:
200m sprint
15 pushups
15 lunges
100m sprint

15 squats

Beginner Workout 17
5 rounds for time:
15 push ups
15 sit ups
15 jump squats

Beginner Workout 18
1 minute plank
500 meter run
2 minute plank
500 meter run
3 minute plank
500m cool down jog

Beginner Workout 19
4 rounds for time:
20 walking lunges
20 push ups
20 jumping jacks

Beginner Workout 20
AMRAP
20 squats
100 meter run
20 walking lunges
10 push ups
10 lunges
100 meter run

Beginner Workout 21
3 rounds for time:
15 vertical jumps
15 jumping jacks
10 burpees
15 push ups

Beginner Workout 22
1 round for time:
skip for 1 minute
20 vertical jumps
20 jumping jacks
skip for 1 minute
20 squats
20 walking lunges

Beginner Workout 23
AMRAP
20 sit ups
20 reverse crunches
20 high knees
20 squat jumps
10 pushups

Beginner Workout 24
7 rounds for time:
7 burpees
7 squats
7 sit ups
7 jumping jacks

Beginner Workout 25
3 rounds for time:
90 second plank
20 burpees
90 second plank
20 vertical jumps

Benchmark – The Girls

'The Girls' are benchmark workouts are designed to measure the improvements in your performance, they are to be performed irregularly.

Angie
For time (complete all reps of each exercise before moving on)
100 pull-ups
100 push-ups
100 sit-ups
100 squats

Barbara
5 rounds for time
20 pull-ups
30 push-ups
40 sit-ups
50 squats

Chelsea
Each minute on the minute for 30 minutes of:
5 pull-ups
10 push-ups
15 squats

Cindy
As many rounds as possible in 20 minutes of:
5 pull-ups
10 push-ups
15 squats

Diane
21-15-9 reps, for time
Deadlift 225lbs
Handstand push-ups

Elizabeth
21-15-9 reps, for time

Clean 135lbs
Ring Dips

Fran
21-15-9 reps, for time
Thruster 95lbs
Pull-ups

Grace
30 reps for time
Clean and jerk 135lbs

Helen
3 rounds for time
400 meter run
1.5 pood kettlebell swing x 21
Pull-ups 12 reps

Isabel
30 reps for time
Snatch 135 pounds

Jackic
For time
1000 meter row
Thruster 45lbs – 50 reps
Pull-ups – 30 reps

Karen
For time
Wall-ball – 150 shots

Linda (aka '3 bars of death')
10/9/8/7/6/5/4/3/2/1 rep rounds for time

Deadlift 1.5 BW
Bench 1x BW
Clean ¾ BW

Mary
As many rounds as possible in 20 minutes of:
5 handstand push-ups
10 1 legged squats
15 pull-ups

Nancy
5 rounds for time
400 meter run
overhead squat 95lbs x 15

Annie
50-40-30-20-10 rep rounds for time
Reps of:
Doubleunders
Sit-ups

Eva
5 rounds for time
Run 800 meters
2 pood KB swing, 30 reps
30 pull-ups

Kelly
Five rounds for time
Run 400 meters
30 box jump, 24 inch box
30 wall ball shots, 20 pound ball

Lynne
5 rounds for max reps (not timed)
Bodyweight bench press (if you weight 170lbs, you will bench 170lbs)
Pull-ups

Nicole
As many rounds as possible in 20 minutes of:
Run 400m
Max rep pull-ups

Benchmark - Hero WODs

The Hero workouts are workouts created in honour of soldiers and law enforcement officers who have fallen while serving for their country. These workouts are not for the faint hearted – they are extremely tough, not designed for beginners. The Heroes, just like The Girls are to be used irregularly for assessing your progress instead of performing the regular WOD.

JT
21-15-9 reps, for time
Handstand push-ups
Ring dips
Push-ups

Michael
3 rounds for time
Run 800 meters
50 back extensions
50 Sit-ups

Murph
For time, partition the pull-ups, push-ups and squats as necessary
1 mile run
100 pull-ups
200 push-ups
300 squats
1 mile run

Daniel
For time
50 pull-ups
400 meter run
95 pound thruster – 21 reps
800 meter run
95 pound thruster – 21 reps
400 meter run
50 pull-ups

Josh
For time
95 pound overhead squat – 21 reps
42 pull-ups
95 pound overhead squat – 15 reps
30 pull-ups
95 pound overhead squats – 9 reps
18 pull-ups

Jason
For time
100 squats
5 muscle-ups
75 squats
10 muscle-ups
50 squats
15 muscle-ups
15 squats
20 muscle-ups

Badger
3 rounds for time
95 pound squat clean – 30 reps
30 pull-ups
Run 800 meters

Joshie
3 rounds for time
40 pound dumbbell snatch – 21 reps right arm
40 pound dumbbell snatch – 21 reps left arm
21 L pull-ups
Note: snatches are full squat snatches

Nate

As many rounds as possible in 20 minutes
2 muscle-ups
4 handstand push-ups
8 2-pood kettlebell swings

Randy

For time

Tommy V

For time
115lb thruster – 21 reps
15ft rope climb – 12 ascents
115lb thruster – 15 reps
15ft rope climb – 12 ascents
115lb thruster – 9 reps
15ft rope climb – 6 ascents

Griff

For time
Run 800 meters
Run 400 meters backwards
Run 800 meters
Run 400 meters backwards

Ryan

For time
five rounds of:
7 muscle-ups
21 burpees
Note: each burpee terminates with a jump one foot above max standing reach

Erin
For time
five rounds of:
40lb dumbbell split clean – 15 reps
21 pull-ups

Mr Joshua
For time
five rounds of:
Run 400 meters
30 glute-ham sit-ups
250lb deadlift – 15 reps

DT
For time
five rounds of:
155lb deadlift – 12 reps
155lb hang power clean – 9 reps
155lb pound push jerk – 6 reps

Danny
Maximum number of rounds in 20 minutes of:
24 inch box jump – 30 reps
115lb push press – 20 reps
30 pull-ups

Hansen
For time
five rounds of:
30 reps – 2 pood kettlebell swing
30 burpees
30 glute-ham sit-ups

Tyler
For time
five rounds of:
7 muscle-ups
95lb Sumo-deadlift high-pulls – 21 reps

Lumberjack 20
For time
20 deadlifts (275lbs)
Run 400m
20 KB swings (2 pood)
Run 400m
20 overhead squats (115lbs)
Run 400m
20 Burpees
Run 400m
20 Pull-ups (Chest to Bar)
Run 400m
20 Box jumps (24")
Run 400m
20 DB Squat Cleans (45lbs each)
Run 400m

Stephen
For time
30-25-15-10-5 rep rounds of:
GHD sit-up
Back extension
Knees to elbow
95lb stiff legged deadlift

Garrett
For time
3 rounds of:
75 squats
25 ring handstand push-ups
25 L-pull-ups

War Frank
For time
3 rounds of:
25 muscle-ups
100 squats
35 GHD sit-ups

McGhee
Rounds in 30 minutes
275lb deadlift – 5 reps
13 push-ups
9 box jumps 24 inch box

Paul
For time
5 rounds of:
50 double unders
35 knees to elbows
185lb overhead walk – 20 yards

Jerry
For time
Run 1 mike
Row 2k
Run 1 mile

Nutts
For time
10 handstand push-ups
250lb deadlift – 15 reps
24 box jumps – 30 inch box
50 pull-ups
100 wallball shots – 20lbs, 10"
200 double-unders
Run 400 meters with a 45lb plate

Arnie
For time
with a single 2 pood kettlebell:
21 Turkish get-ups – right arm
50 swings
21 overhead squats – left arm
50 swings
21 overhead squats – right arm
50 swings
21 Turkish get-ups – left arm

The Seven
For time
Seven rounds of:
7 handstand push-ups
135lb thruster – 7 reps
7 knees to elbows
245lb deadlift – 7 reps
7 burpees
7 Kettlebell swings – 2 pood
7 pull-ups

RJ
For time
five rounds of:
Run 800 meters
15ft rope climb – 5 ascents
50 push-ups

Luce
For time
wearing a 20lb vest, perform 3 rounds of:
run 1K
10 muscle-ups
100 squats

Johnson
Rounds in 20 minutes
245lb deadlift – 9 reps
8 muscle-ups
155lb squat clean – 9 reps

Roy
For time
five rounds of:
225lb deadlift – 15 reps
20 box jumps – 24 inch box
25 pull-ups

Adam Brown
For time
two rounds of:
295lb deadlift – 24 reps
24 box jumps – 24 inch box
24 wallball shots – 20lb ball

195lb bench press – 24 reps
24 box jumps – 24 inch box
24 wallball shots – 20lb ball
145lb clean – 24 reps

Coe
For time
ten rounds of:
95lb thruster – 10 reps
10 ring push-ups

Severin
For time
50 strict pull-ups
100 push-ups release hands from floor at the bottom
Run 5k
Note: wear 20lb weighted vest if possible

Helton
For time
3 rounds of:
Run 800 meters
50lb dumbbell squat cleans - 30 reps
30 burpees

Jack
Max rounds in 20 minutes
115lb push press – 10 reps
1.5 pood KB swings – 10 swings
10 box jumps 24 inch box

Forrest
For time
3 rounds of:
20 L-pull-ups
30 toes to bar
40 burpees
800 meter run

Bulger
For time
Ten rounds of:
Run 150 meters
chest to bar pull-ups – 7 reps
135lb front squat – 7 reps
Handstand push-ups – 7 reps

Brenton
For time
Five rounds of:
Bear crawl 100 feet
Standing broad-jump – 100 feet
Note: wear 20lb weighted vest if possible

Blake
For time
4 rounds of:
100 foot walking lunge with 45lb plate held overhead
30 box jumps – 24 inch box
20 wallball shots – 20lb ball
10 handstand push-ups

Colin
For time
6 rounds of:
Carry 50lb sandbag 400 meters
115lb push press – 12 reps
12 box jumps – 24 inch box
95lb sumo deadlift high-pull – 12 reps

Thompson
For time
10 rounds of:
15ft rope climb – 1 ascent
95lb back squat – 29 reps
135lb barbells farmer carry – 10 meters
Note: begin the rope climbs seated on the floor

Whitten
For time
5 rounds of:
22 kettlebell swings – 2 pood
22 box jumps – 24 inch box
run 400 meters
22 burpees
22 wall ball shots – 20lb ball

Bull
For time
2 rounds of:
200 double-unders
135lb overhead squat -50 reps
50 pull-ups
run 1 mile

Rankel
AMRAP – 20 minutes
225lb deadlift – 6 reps
burpee pull-ups – 7 reps
2 pood KB swings – 10 swings
run 200 meters

Holbrook
Each round for time
Ten rounds of:
115lb thruster – 5 reps
10 pull-ups
100 meter sprint
1 minute rest

Ledesma
AMRAP – 20 minutes
5 parallette handstand push-ups
10 toes through rings
20 pound medicine ball cleans – 15 reps

Wittman
For time
7 rounds of:
1.5 pood KB swings – 15 swings
95lb power clean – 15 reps
15 box jumps – 24 inch box

Mccluskey
For time
3 rounds of:
9 muscle-ups
15 burpee pull-ups

21 pull-ups
run 800 meters

Weaver
For time
4 rounds of:
10 L-pull-ups
15 push-ups
15 chest to bar pull-ups
15 push-ups
20 pull-ups
15 push-ups

Abbate
For time
Run 1 mile
155lb clean and jerk – 21 reps
run 800 meters
155lb clean and jerk – 21 reps
Run 1 mile

Hammer
Each round for time
135lb power clean – 5 reps
135lb front squat – 10 reps
135lb jerk – 5 reps
20 pull-ups
Note: rest for 90 seconds between rounds

Moore
Rounds in 20 minutes
15ft rope climb – 1 ascent
run 400 meters
max rep handstand push-ups

Wilmot
For time
6 rounds of:
50 squats
25 ring dips

Moon
For time
7 rounds of:
40lb dumbbell hang split snatch – 10 reps right arm
15ft rope climb – 1 ascent
40lb dumbbell hang split snatch – 10 reps left arm
15ft rope climb – 1 ascent
Note: alternate feet in the split snatch sets

Small
For time
3 rounds of:
row 1000 meters
50 burpees
50 box jumps – 24 inch box
run 800 meters

Bodyweight WODs

The following WODs are based entirely around bodyweight exercises, these are broken down into several sub-categories based on the equipment required e.g. pull-up bar, rings and skipping rope.

Workouts - No Equipment Required

No Equip WOD 1
Walking lunges for 400m

No Equip WOD 2
150 burpees

No Equip WOD 3
4 rounds of:
Run 400m
50 squats
100-75-50-25 reps:
situps
flutterkicks
Leg levers

No Equip WOD 4
50 burpees

No Equip WOD 5
Cumulative L-hold for 5 minutes
Use a bar, rings, or floor

No Equip WOD 6
50 squats
25 pushups
50 pistol squats
25 fingertip pushups
50 side lunges
25 knuckle pushups
50 walking lunges
25 diamond pushups

No Equip WOD 7
50 flutterkicks
50 situps
Run 400m
100 flutterkicks
100 situps
Run 400m

No Equip WOD 8
20-16-12-8-4 reps of:
One-arm pushups
Pistol squats

No Equip WOD 9
4 rounds of:
50 pushups
50 situps
50 flutterkicks

No Equip WOD 10
1 round Tabata sprints (8 rounds, 20 seconds on, 10 seconds off)
1 round Tabata bottom-to-bottom squats (8 rounds, 20 seconds on, 10 seconds off)

No Equip WOD 11
AMRAP in 12 minutes of:
10 pushups
15 situps
20m walking lunge

No Equip WOD 12
21-15-9 reps of:
lunges
situps
burpees

No Equip WOD 13
5 rounds of:
50 mountain climbers
25 situps

No Equip WOD 14
5 rounds of:
100 jumping jacks
100 mountain climbers

No Equip WOD 15
Burpees: 20-19-18-17 ...4- 3-2-1
Walk 25m after each set

No Equip WOD 16
50 rounds of:
1 squat
1 pushup
1 situp
1 superman
1 tuck jump

No Equip WOD 17
50 jumping jacks
50 pushups
50 tuck jumps
50 situps

50 mountain climbers
50 squats
50 jumping jacks

No Equip WOD 18
10 rounds:
30 second handstand
30 second isometric squat

No Equip WOD 19
Run 100m
20 pushups
5 burpees
15 clap pushups
5 burpees
10 chest-slap pushups
5 burpees
5 fingertip pushups
Run 100m
15 pushups
5 burpees
10 clap pushups
5 burpees
10 chest-slap pushups
5 burpees
5 fingertip pushups
Run 100m
10 pushups
5 burpees
10 clap pushups

No Equip WOD 20
5 burpees
10 chest-slap pushups

5 burpees
5 fingertip pushups

No Equip WOD 21
Run 400m
Burpee-Broad Jump 25m
Walking Lunges 25m
Burpee-Broad Jump 25m
Bear Crawl 25m
Burpee-Broad Jump 25m
Walking Lunges 25m
Burpee-Broad Jump 25m
Bear Crawl 25m
Run 400m

No Equip WOD 22
100 situps
100 flutterkicks
100 leg levers

No Equip WOD 23
Use a deck of cards:
Face cards= 10
Aces = 11
Numbered cards are as per number states
Flip each card and perform the movement and the number of reps specified
WOD is complete once the whole deck has been utilised
Hearts - burpees
Diamonds – mountain climbers
Spades - flutterkicks
Clubs - situps
Jokers - Run 400m

No Equip WOD 24
50 burpees
75 flutterkicks
100 pushups
150 situps

No Equip WOD 25
5 rounds:
10 burpees
20 box jumps
30 pushups
40 squats
50 lunges

No Equip WOD 26
4 rounds:
50 walking lunges
50 squats
Run 400m

No Equip WOD 27
Run 5km
Stop every 120 seconds to perform 20 pushups, 20 situps and 20 squats

No Equip WOD 28
3 rounds:
50 pushups
50 situps
50 squats

No Equip WOD 29
5 rounds:
50 walking lunges
15 handstand pushups
80 squats
10 handstand pushups
60 squats
20 handstand pushups
40 squats
30 handstand pushups
20 squats

No Equip WOD 30
4 rounds:
25 lunges
50 squats
5 rounds of:
100 squats
20 lunges
35 pushups

No Equip WOD 31
5 rounds of:
50 squats
30 handstand pushups

No Equip WOD 32
2 rounds:
Max pushups in 2 minutes
Max situps in 2 minutes
Max flutterkicks in 2 minutes
Max squats in 2 minutes

No Equip WOD 33
3 rounds of:
30 yard bear crawl
30 yard inch worm pushup
30 yard burpee jumps

Workouts - Pullup Bar Required

No Equip WOD 34
100 burpee pullups

No Equip WOD 35
AMRAP in 20 minutes of:
15 pullups
30 pushups
45 squats

No Equip WOD 36
1 round:
Handstand pushups: 15-13-11-9-7-5-3-1
L-pullups: 1-3-5-7-9-11-13-15

No Equip WOD 37
3 rounds:
Run 800m
50 pullups

No Equip WOD 38
10 rounds:
12 burpees
12 pullups

No Equip WOD 39
5 rounds:
15 L-pullups
30 pushups
45 situps

No Equip WOD 40
5 rounds:
25 inverted burpees
25 pullups
25 burpees

No Equip WOD 41
30 handstand pushups
10 pullups
20 handstand pushups
20 pullups
10 handstand pushups
30 pullups

No Equip WOD 42
Run 800m
40 L-pullups
Run 800m
40 strict pullups
Run 800m
40 kipping pullups

No Equip WOD 43
5 rounds of:
50 squats
30 pullups
15 handstand pushups
100 squats
100 pullups
200 pushups
300 squats
100 lunges

No Equip WOD 44
21-15-9 reps of:
burpees
pullups

No Equip WOD 45
21-15-9 reps of:
pullups
pushups
squat jumps to 14" above max reach

No Equip WOD 46
50-35-20 rep rounds of:
handstand pushups
pullups

No Equip WOD 47
AMRAP in 15 minutes:
20 seconds of pullups
20 seconds of situps
20 seconds of squats

No Equip WOD 48
100 pullups
200 pushups
300 squats
50 situps

No Equip WOD 49
AMRAP in 20 minutes of:
25 pullups
50 pushups
75 squats

No Equip WOD 50
AMRAP in 20 minutes of:
25 handstand pushups
50 pistol squats
75 pullups

No Equip WOD 51
AMRAP in 20 minutes of:
10 L pullups
20 squats

No Equip WOD 52
Run 1600M
100 bodyblasters (burpee-pullups-knees to elbows)
Run 1600M

No Equip WOD 53
Tabata pullups, 1 round
Run 1600m
Tabata pushups, 1 round
Run 1600m
Tabata situps, 1 round
Run 1600m
Tabata squats, 1 round
Run 1600m

No Equip WOD 54
10-20-30 reps of:
squat
handstand pushups
squat
pullups

No Equip WOD 55
100 pullups
Run 1 mile
100 pushups
Run 1 mile
100 situps
Run 1 mile
100 squats
Run 1 mile

No Equip WOD 56
Run 1 mile
50 pullups
100 pushups
150 situps
200 squats
Run 1 mile
50 pullups
100 pushups
150 situps
200 squats
Run 1 mile

No Equip WOD 57
5 rounds of:
30 handstand pushups
30 pullups

No Equip WOD 58
100 squats
20 handstand pushups
30 pullups
100 squats

9 handstand pushups
200 squats
15 handstand pushups
100 squats
21 handstand pushups

No Equip WOD 59
100 L-pullups
100 squats
40 pullups
80 squats
32 pullups
60 squats
24 pullups
40 squats
16 pullups
20 squats
8 pullups

No Equip WOD 60
10 rounds of:
10 pullups
20 pushups
30 squats

No Equip WOD 61
AMRAP in 20 minutes of:
7 handstand pushups
12 L-pullups

No Equip WOD 62
50 squats
50 pullups

50 walking lunges
50 knees-to-elbows
5 handstand pushups
50 situps
5 handstand pushups
50 squats
50 pullups

No Equip WOD 63
100 squats
25 situps
100 squats
25 situps
100 squats
25 knees-to-elbows
100 squats
25 handstand pushups

No Equip WOD 64
2 rounds of:
35 squats
35 knees-to-elbows
35 squats
35 situps
35 lunges
35 squats

No Equip WOD 65
21-18-15-12-9-6-3 of:
squats
L-pullups
knees-to-elbows

No Equip WOD 66
7 rounds of:
35 squats
25 pushups
15 pullups

No Equip WOD 67
21-15-9 reps of:
Body blasters (burpee-pullup-knees to elbows)
box jump burpees
Belushi burpees (on jump turn 180 degrees)
Burpee Jacks (plank jack to jumping jack)

No Equip WOD 68
3 rounds of:
100 squats
25 L-pullups
30 handstand pushups
5 rounds of:
9 handstand pushups
9 pullups

No Equip WOD 69
21 pullups
50 squats
21 knees-to-elbows
18 pullups
50 squats
18 knees-to-elbows
15 pullups
50 squats
15 knees-to-elbows
12 pullups

50 squats
12 knees-to-elbows

No Equip WOD 70
20 rounds of:
5 pullups
5 pushups
5 situps
5 squats

No Equip WOD 71
100 squats
21 handstand pushups
30 pullups
100 squats
30 pullups
21 handstand pushups
100 squats

No Equip WOD 72
5 rounds of:
20 squats
20 pushups
20 pullups

No Equip WOD 73
50-40-30-20-10 reps
pullups
squat jumps

No Equip WOD 74
15 rounds for max reps:
Pullups - 30 seconds on 20 seconds off

No Equip WOD 75
100 squats
20 handstand pushups
30 pullups
100 squats
30 pullups
20 handstand pushups
100 squats

No Equip WOD 76
Run 400m
25 pullups
25 pushups
25 situps
25 squats

No Equip WOD 77
150 squats
50 pushups
21 pullups
Run 800m
21 pullups
50 pushups
150 squats

No Equip WOD 78
50 L-pullups
50 handstand pushups
50 pistol squats
50 knees-to-elbows

No Equip WOD 79
3 rounds of:
Run 800m
30 burpees
30 knees-to-elbows

No Equip WOD 80
21-15-9 reps of:
handstand pushups
Inverted pullups

No Equip WOD 81
20 Burpee Pullups
Run 800m
20 Burpee Pullups
Run 800m
20 Burpee Pullups

Workouts – Rings & Pullup Bar Required

No Equip WOD 82
50-40-30-20-10 reps of:
Pullups
Ring dips

No Equip WOD 83
7 rounds of:
10 pistols squats
12 ring dips
15 pullups

No Equip WOD 84
30 muscle-ups

No Equip WOD 85
50 ring dips
Run 400m
50 pushups
Run 400m
50 handstand pushups
Run 400m

No Equip WOD 86
Use a timer:
1 muscle-up the first minute
2 muscle-ups the second minute
3 muscle-ups the third minute
Run 400m
Repeat ladder for deadhang pullups
Run 400m
Repeat ladder for kipping pullups
Run 400m

No Equip WOD 87
1 ring dip the first minute
2 ring dips the second minute
3 ring dips the third minute
4 ring dips the fourth minute
Continue until failure

No Equip WOD 88
50 ring dips
100 squats
50 ring dips
100 squats
50 ring dips

No Equip WOD 89
5 rounds of:
Max ring dips in 60 seconds
60 seconds recovery
Max ring pushups in 60 seconds
60 seconds recovery

No Equip WOD 90
5 rounds of:
Max rep ring dips
Max rep pullups

No Equip WOD 91
4 rounds of:
50 squats
5 muscle-ups

No Equip WOD 92
100 squats
30 muscle-ups
100 squats

No Equip WOD 93
3 rounds of:
100 squats
50 ring dips
30 L-pullups

No Equip WOD 94
3 rounds of:
100 squats
20 ring pushups
12 pullups

No Equip WOD 95
5 rounds of:
50 squats
15 ring pushups

No Equip WOD 96
10-9-8-7-6-5-4-3-2-1
pullups
ring pushups
handstand pushups

No Equip WOD 97
2 rounds of:
21 lunges
21 pullups
21 squats

21 ring dips
21 handstand pushups

No Equip WOD 98
AMRAP in 20 minutes:
10 False grip ring pullups
10 ring dips

No Equip WOD 99
7 rounds of:
20 ring dips
20 pullups
20 lunges

No Equip WOD 100
10 rounds of:
10 L-pull ups
10 ring pushups
10 knees-to-elbows

No Equip WOD 101
10 ring pushups
10 Archer pushups
10 ring flies
10 wide grip ring pushups
10 Single leg ring pushups
10 Pseudo planche ring pushups
10 Jack-knife ring pushups
10 Dive Bomber ring pushups
10 Elevated ring pushups
10 ring pushups

No Equip WOD 102
25 handstand pushups
25 squats
25 pullups
25 pistols
25 muscle-ups

No Equip WOD 103
3 rounds of:
100 squats
50 ring dips

No Equip WOD 104
4 rounds of:
5 muscle-ups
50 straight-leg lifts on rings

No Equip WOD 105
AMRAP in 20 minutes of:
10 pullups
10 ring dips
10 walking lunges

No Equip WOD 106
5 rounds of:
5 handstand pushups
5 muscle-ups

No Equip WOD 107
3 rounds of:
7 muscle-ups
100 squats

No Equip WOD 108
120 pullups and 120 ring dips
Partition if necessary

No Equip WOD 109
5 rounds of:
10 ring dips
15 pullups
20 handstand pushups

No Equip WOD 110
25 squats
25 situps
25 lunges
25 handstand pushups
25 pushups
25 knees-to-elbows
25 ring dips
25 pullups

No Equip WOD 111
50 squats
50 jumping pullups
50 steps walking lunge
50 knees-to-elbows
50 handstand pushups
50 situps
50 ring dips
50 squats
50 pushups

No Equip WOD 112
Run 1 mile
60 push ups
40 ring dips
20 handstand pushups
10 pistol squats
20 handstand pushups
40 ring dips
60 push ups
Run 1 mile

No Equip WOD 113
Ladder for 45 minutes:
Pullups by 1
Ring dips by 2
Pushups by 3
Situps by 3

No Equip WOD 114
100 burpees
100 handstand pushups
100 pullups
100 ring dips
100 ring rows
100 pushups
100 windshield wipers
100 situps
100 knees to elbows
100 flutterkicks

No Equip WOD 115
3 rounds – 120 seconds rest between rounds:
50 squats
30 pullups
40 pushups
50 squats

No Equip WOD 116
Run 1 mile
30 pullups
60 pushups

No Equip WOD 117
5 rounds of:
50 squats
21 ring dips
21 handstand pushups

Workouts – Skipping Rope, Bar, Rings Required

No Equip WOD 115
3 rounds – 90 second intervals of:
burpees
pushups
box/bench jumps
pullups
Double Unders
squats

No Equip WOD 116
90 seconds of skipping
50 lunges
50 pushups
50 situps
90 seconds of skipping
40 lunges
40 pushups
40 situps
90 seconds of skipping
30 lunges
30 pushups
30 situps
90 seconds of skipping
20 lunges
20 pushups
20 situps
90 seconds of skipping
10 lunges
10 pushups
10 situps

No Equip WOD 117
5 rounds of:
50 squats
100 rope jumps

No Equip WOD 118
100 rope jumps
21 knees-to-elbows
50 Push ups
15 L-Pull ups
100 rope jumps
15 knees-to-elbows
35 Push ups
12 L-Pull ups
100 rope jumps
12 knees-to-elbows
20 Push ups
9 L-Pull ups

No Equip WOD 119
4 rounds of:
100 jump ropes
Run 400 meters
10 Bodyblasters (burpee-pullup-knees-toelbows)

No Equip WOD 120
50 situps
50 double-unders
50 situps
50 walking lunges
50 situps
50 burpees
50 situps

No Equip WOD 121
50-30-20 reps of:
double-unders
pushups
pullups
3 rounds of:
50 double-unders
75 squats

Running WODs

The following workouts are entirely based around sprints and distance running, these WODs are designed to improve cardiovascular health as well as increase your speed and agility.

Running WOD 1
2 mile run for best time

Running WOD 2
Max distance in 30 minutes

Running WOD 3
1 round Tabata uphill sprints (20:10 x 8)

Running WOD 4
4 rounds of:
5:00 max distance
3:00 recovery

Running WOD 5
3 rounds:
5km run with 30 second recovery between rounds

Running WOD 6
1.2km uphill sprint
Rest 1:00
1.2km downhill jog
Rest 1:00
Repeat

Running WOD 7
1:00 sprint, 1:00 rest
1:00 sprint, 0:50 rest
1:00 sprint, 0:40 rest
1:00 sprint, 0:30 rest
1:00 sprint, 0:20 rest
1:00 sprint, 0:10 rest
1:00 sprint, 0:20 rest

1:00 sprint, 0:30 rest
1:00 sprint, 0:40 rest
1:00 sprint, 0:50 rest
1:00 sprint, 1:00 rest

Running WOD 8
10x100m with 2:00 rest
8x200m with 2:00 rest
4x400m with 5:00 rest
8 rounds of:
80 second sprint, 40 second rest

Running WOD 9
3 rounds of:
1:00 sprint, 1:00 recovery
2:00 sprint, 2:00 recovery
3:00 sprint, 3:00 recovery

Running WOD 10
3:00 sprint, 3:00 recovery
2:00 sprint, 2:00 recovery
1:00 sprint, 1:00 recovery
2:00 sprint, 2:00 recovery
3:00 sprint, 3:00 recovery

Running WOD 11
4x800m with 2:00 rest
Run 10k. Run second half faster than the first.

Running WOD 12
3 rounds of:
100m sprint, Rest same amount of time you finished the sprint
200m sprint, Rest same amount of time you finished the sprint
300m sprint, Rest same amount of time you finished the sprint

Running WOD 13
3 rounds of:
200m sprint, Rest same amount of time you finished the sprint
400m sprint, Rest same amount of time you finished the sprint
600m sprint, Rest same amount of time you finished the sprint

Running WOD 15
10 rounds of:
1:00 sprint, 1:00 recovery

Running WOD 16
8 rounds of:
10 seconds sprint, 5 seconds recovery

Running WOD 17
0:45 sprint, 0:45 recovery
1:30 sprint, 1:30 recovery
3:00 sprint, 3:00 recovery
6:00 sprint, 6:00 recovery
3:00 sprint, 3:00 recovery
1:30 sprint, 1:30 recovery
0:45 sprint, 0:45 recovery

Running WOD 18
16 rounds of:
10 seconds sprint, 20 seconds recovery

Running WOD 19
4x200m + 4x400m + 2x1000m
Rest 1:00, 1:30, and 2:00 per interval distance, respectively.

Running WOD 20
200m sprint, Rest same amount of time you finished the sprint
400m sprint, Rest same amount of time you finished the sprint
600m sprint, Rest same amount of time you finished the sprint
400m sprint, Rest same amount of time you finished the sprint
200m sprint, Rest same amount of time you finished the sprint

Running WOD 21
1 mile time trial
Rest 60 seconds
2x400m sprint
Rest 60 seconds between sprints

Running WOD 22
4x200m
2x400m
Rest 60 seconds between sprints

C2 Rowing WODs

The following WODs are entirely rowing based, specifically on a C2 rowing machine.
These workouts are designed to increase your cardiovascular health and fitness as well as your speed and agility.

C2 WOD 1
Time trial
Row 1500m
Set damper setting to 10

C2 WOD 2
Intervals
For total distance
Row 9x (60:60)

C2 WOD 3
Intervals
Cover max distance
Row 6x (90:90)

C2 WOD 4
Intervals
For max distance
Row 20 (15:10)

C2 WOD 5
Intervals
Record average time for all intervals
Row 10x250m
Rest for 5x interval time

C2 WOD 6
5 rounds
Partner effort, one rows while the other recovers
Row 50-40-30-20-10 calories

C2 WOD 7
Time trial
Row 4000m

C2 WOD 8
Intervals
Row 4x1200m
Rest 2 minutes between intervals

C2 WOD 9
Intervals
Rest 45 seconds between intervals
Row 8x250m

C2 WOD 10
5 rounds
Row for total distance or calories
10:10
20:10
10:10
30:10
15:10
25:60

C2 WOD 11
Intervals
For total distance
Row 9x (60:60)

C2 WOD 12
Intervals
Row 6x (90:90)

C2 WOD 13
Intervals
Row 3x2500m
Rest 1 minute between intervals

C2 WOD 14
Intervals
2 rounds, cover max distance
Row 1 minute
Rest 1 minute
Row 1 minute
Rest 50 seconds
Row 1 minute
Rest 40 seconds
Row 1 minute
Rest 30 seconds
Row 1 minute
Rest 20 seconds
Row 1 minute
Rest 10 seconds

C2 WOD 15
3 rounds
Your calories spent is your score
Row 2 minutes
Rest 3 minutes
Row 1 minute, arms only
Rest 1 minute
Row 1 minute
Rest 3 minutes

Kettlebell WODs

The following WODs are based around kettlebells – ranging from WODs that require a single kettlebell to WODs that require a matching pair of kettlebells.

Ensure you are using kettlebell(s) of an appropriate weight to avoid injury.

KB WOD 1
2 rounds:
50x Kettlebell Hand-to-hand swings
25x Kettlebell Double bottoms-up press
12x Kettlebell Snatch
50x Push-ups

KB WOD 2
For time:
Run 1 mile
100x KB snatch
200x Alternating KB press
300x KB swing
Run 1 mile

KB WOD 3
18 rounds:
1-2-3-2-3-4-3-4-5-4-5-6-5-6-7-6-7-8x reps
Double clean
Jerk

KB WOD 4
For time:
40x Plyo push-ups using KB handles
40x Hanging guard sit-ups
40x Pull-ups
40x Bench press
40x KB swing
40x Alternating KB press
Row 50 calories

KB WOD 5
AMRAP in 10 minutes:
1x Double KB snatch
2x KB Sotts press
3x KB thrusters
4x Push-ups

KB WOD 6
For max rounds:
On-the-minute Double KB Sumo deadlift
Start at 1 rep, add another rep at top of each minute
Continue until you cannot perform the requisite number of reps per round

KB WOD 7
Max reps in 10 minutes
Switch arms as necessary, KB may not touch floor
Long cycle KB clean & jerk

KB WOD 8
1 round:
Row 2km
200x KB swings
Row 2000m

KB WOD 9
8 rounds:
8x Single arm KB thruster
8x Pistol squats
8x KB reverse lunge

KB WOD 10
13 rounds:
21-18-15-12-9-6-3-6-9-12-15-18-21x reps
KB swings
Push-ups

KB WOD 11
3 rounds - 21-15-9x reps:
KB sumo high-pull
Double KB push jerk

KB WOD 12
AMRAP in 12 minutes:
3x KB pistol squats
6x Double KB snatch
9x KB jerk

KB WOD 13
Max rounds:
On the minute every minute perform
1x KB snatch first minute, then rest
2x KB snatch second minute, then rest
3x KB snatch third minute...
Continue until failure

KB WOD 14
18 rounds:
1-2-3-2-3-4-3-4-5-4-5-6-5-6-7-6-7-8x reps
Double snatch
Thruster

KB WOD 15
Max rounds:
On-the-minute Double KB Snatch
Start at 1 rep, add another rep at top of each minute
Continue until you cannot perform the requisite number of reps per round

KB WOD 16
For time:
Use single KB
25x Ring dips
25x Walking lunges w/ KB overhead
50x Hand-to-hand swing
25x Walking lunges w/ KB overhead
50x Pull-ups
25x Ring dips

KB WOD 17
Max rounds in 12 minutes:
7x KB snatch
7x Ball slams
7x GHD sit-ups

KB WOD 18
5 rounds:
KB swings 80-40-20-40-80x
Push-ups 40-20-10-20-40x
Pull-ups 20-10-5-10-20x

KB WOD 19
3 rounds:
21-15-9x reps

KB sumo high-pull
Double KB push jerk

KB WOD 20
Max rounds in 7 minutes:
3x Back squat (bw)
6x Double KB swing (1/2 bw)
9x Push-ups

KB WOD 21
5 rounds:
20x Hand to hand KB swing
10x Double KB clean
20x Alternating bent KB row
10x Thruster

KB WOD 22
3 rounds:
5x Double KB snatch
10x Thrusters
20x Renegade rows

KB WOD 23
5 rounds:
All exercises are double KB
6x Front squat
6x Clean
6x Press
15x Swing
6x Bent row
10x Burpees

KB WOD 24
Max rounds in 20 minutes;
3x KB snatch, each arm
5x Burpees

KB WOD 25
10 rounds:
6x KB snatch, each arm

KB WOD 26
4 rounds:
10-20-30-40x reps
KB swing
Man-makers
Alternating floor press

KB WOD 27
For max distance:
KB Farmer's walk for 12 minutes
Stop at top of each minute and do 5x burpees

KB WOD 28
3 rounds:
21-15-9x reps
KB thrusters
Ring pull-ups

KB WOD 29
For time:
75x KB snatch

KB WOD 30
For time:
53x KB swing
53x KB sumo deadlift high-pull
53x KB snatch
53x KB back extension

KB WOD 31
Max rounds in 15 minutes;
10x KB suitcase deadlift
Farmer's walk - 20 steps

KB WOD 32
For time:
20x KB swing
30x Single KB thruster, left arm
20x Push-ups
30x Sit-ups
20x KB sumo deadlift high pull
30x Burpees
20x Double KB snatch
200m Farmer's walk
20x KB swing

KB WOD 33
29 rounds:
Breathing ladder
KB swing

KB WOD 34
3 rounds:
5x Burpees
10x KB thrusters

15x KB sumo deadlift high-pull
20x Sit-ups

KB WOD 35
For time:
Use single KB
25x Ring dips
25x Walking lunges w/ KB overhead (left arm)
50x Hand-to-hand swing
25x Walking lunges w/ KB overhead (right arm)
50x Pull-ups
25x Ring dips

KB WOD 36
Max rounds in 12 minutes:
3x Clean
3x Front squat
3x Double Snatch
3x Bent row

KB WOD 37
5 rounds:
21x Sumo deadlift high pull
21x Burpees
Row 250m

KB WOD 38
3 rounds:
5x Double KB sumo deadlift
10x KB Goblet squat
40m Overhead carry
25x KB swings

KB WOD 39
3 rounds:
6x KB turkish get-up
6x KB clean/press/windmill combo
50m Heavy sandbag carry

KB WOD 40
For time:
Use two KBs for all weighted movements.
12x KB swing
12x Snatch
12x Clean & jerk
12x Bent rows
12x Burpees
12x High pulls
12x Mountain climbers
12x Sotts press
12x Suitcase swings
12x Push-ups on KB handles

KB WOD 41
3 rounds:
15x KB swings
15x each arm KB clean & jerk
15x KB goblet squats
30 KB Hand-to-hand swings
15x each arm KB snatch

KB WOD 42
Max rounds in 15 minutes:
Use single KB for all movements, KB may not touch floor
1x Snatch
1x Overhead squat

1x Windmill
1x Jerk
1x Hand-to-hand swing

KB WOD 43
For time:
400m KB Farmer's walk
50x Bottoms-up single KB thruster
25x/arm KB snatch
50x Alternating floor press
400m KB Farmer's walk

KB WOD 44
3 rounds:
KB snatch intervals, count total reps for score
10:10
20:10
10:10
30:10
15:10
25:60

KB WOD 45
For time:
Use single KB
25x Ring dips
25x Walking lunges w/ KB overhead (left arm)
50x Hand-to-hand swing
25x Walking lunges w/ KB overhead (right arm)
50x Pull-ups
25x Ring dips

KB WOD 46
For time:
50x reps of the following KB complex:
1x Snatch + 1x Push-press + 1x Reverse TGU + 1x Hand-to-hand swing

KB WOD 47
3 rounds:
Double unders 42-30-18x reps
KB swings 21-15-9x reps

KB WOD 48
10 rounds:
KB Snatch 10-9-8-7-6-5-4-3-2-1x
Burpee 1-2-3-4-5-6-7-8-9-10x
KB thruster 10-9-8-7-6-5-4-3-2-1x

KB WOD 49
5 rounds:
20x Hand to hand KB swing
10x Double KB clean
20x Alternating bent KB row
10x Thruster

KB WOD 50
3 rounds:
21-15-9x
Knees to elbows
KB Turkish get-ups
Sit-ups
KB swings
Ring push-ups

KB WOD 51
AMRAP in 12 minutes:
3x Clean
3x Front squat
3x Double Snatch
3x Bent row

KB WOD 52
1 round:
Keep KB off the ground for the entire workout
200x KB swings
150x KB snatch
100x 1-arm KB press

KB WOD 53
Utilise 2 KBs for the following workout:
10x Front squat
20x Alternating bent row
10x Push press
10x Snatch

KB WOD 54
9x KB suitcase deadlift
12x/arm KB snatch
15x KB push press

KB WOD 55
30x KB front squat
30x Push-ups
10x KB snatch
10x Pull-ups, strict

Olympic Lifting WODs

The following WODs are based around Olympic lifts such as the squat, bench press, clean & jerk and snatch. These WODs are designed to increase overall strength & explosive power.

Oly WOD 1
Max rounds:
Rest 60 seconds between rounds, increase weight each round
2x Overhead squat

Oly WOD 2
1 round:
Rest as needed between reps
Sumo deadlift 5-5-3-3-3x

Oly WOD 3
Max rounds:
Perform every minute on the minute, add additional weight on each set
2x Front squat

Oly WOD 4
For time:
Bar may not be set down, rest load on thighs or in hip crease as needed
100x Hang power clean

Oly WOD 5
1 round:
Bar may not be set down, rest load on thighs or in hip crease
100x Hang power clean

Oly WOD 6
Work up to a max load, rest exactly 2 minutes between lifts
Snatch grip deadlift 1RM

Oly WOD 7
5 rounds:
Rest as needed between lifts
Snatch balance 1-1-1-1-1x

Oly WOD 8
Rest as needed between efforts
Snatch deadlift 3-3-3-3x
Front squat 2-2-2-2-2x

Oly WOD 9
5 rounds:
Rest as needed between rounds
Shoulder press 5-5-3-3-1x

Oly WOD 10
Rest as needed between efforts
Snatch 2-2-2-2x
Jerk 2-2-2-2-2x
Clean high pull from blocks 3-3-3x
Back squat 2-2-2-2x

Oly WOD 11
5 rounds:
Rest as needed between rounds
Back squat 5-5-3-3-1x

Oly WOD 12
5 rounds:
Rest as needed between lifts
Squat clean 1-1-1-1-1x

Oly WOD 13
Rest as needed between efforts
Power clean 3-3-3-3-3x
Push press 3-3-3-3-3x

Oly WOD 14
1 round:
Bar may not be set down, rest load on thighs if necessary
100x Hang power clean

Oly WOD 15
For time:
30x Behind-the-neck thrusters

Oly WOD 16
5 rounds:
Rest as needed between lifts
Split jerk 1-1-1-1-1x reps

Oly WOD 17
5 rounds:
Rest as needed between lifts
KB press 5-5-3-3-3x per arm

Oly WOD 18
For time:
30x Clean & jerk
After each lockout rotate 360 degrees with bar in the overhead position

Oly WOD 19
5 rounds:
Rest as needed between lifts
Deadlift 5-5-3-3-1x reps

Oly WOD 20
5 rounds:
Rest as needed between lifts
Overhead squat 3-3-3-3-3x

Oly WOD 21
Heavy singles:
rest as needed between efforts
Snatch 1-1-1-1-1x
Clean & jerk 1-1-1-1-1x
Back squat 1-1-1-1-1x

Oly WOD 22
Rest as needed between efforts
Power snatch 3-3-3-3-3x
Jerk 3-3-3-3-3x
Clean high pull from floor 4-4-4-4-4x
Back squat 8-8-8-6-6x

Oly WOD 23
Tabata 8x (20 seconds work, 10 seconds recovery)
Altlas stone ground to shoulder

Oly WOD 24
Max rounds:
Perform every minute on the minute, add additional weight each round
2x Front squat

Oly WOD 25
For time:
52x Clean & jerk

Oly WOD 26
Rest as needed between sets:
Weighted pull-ups 1-1-1-1-1-1-1x

Oly WOD 27
1-10-1 ladder, teams of two, bar may not be set down until all reps completed
Deadlift

Oly WOD 28
Max reps in 10 minutes:
Switch arms as necessary, KB may not touch floor
Long cycle KB clean & jerk

Oly WOD 29
For time:
30x Clean & jerk (bw)

Oly WOD 30
Max rounds:
Perform one set every minute on the minute, add additional weight until failure
2x Back squat

Strongman WODs

The following WODs are comprised of strongman based exercises and movements.
Be sure to go as heavy as you confidently can on these WODs.

Strongman WOD 1
AMRAP in 12 minutes:
100ft Farmers walk
12x KB swings

Strongman WOD 2
5 rounds:
100ft Farmers walk
10x Handstand push-ups

Strongman WOD 3
AMRAP in 15 minutes:
3x Back squat
2x Muscle-up
1x Atlas stone ground to shoulder (bw)

Strongman WOD 4
Work up to 1RM with as many sets as required:
Front squat
Back squat

Strongman WOD 5
5 rounds:
1-2-3-4-5x Tire flip (3x bw)
5-4-3-2-1x Atlas stone ground to shoulder (bw)

Strongman WOD 6
5 rounds:
5x Log clean and press
50ft Duck walk

Strongman WOD 7
For time:
400m Zercher yoke carry (1.5x bw)

Strongman WOD 8
10 rounds:
50ft Farmers walk
50ft Yoke carry
Rest 1 minute

Strongman WOD 9
Every minute on the minute for max rounds:
1x Jerk
Add additional weight each successive minute, continue until failure

Strongman WOD 10
5 rounds:
30x GHD sit-ups
100ft Farmers walk
10x Tire flips (3x bw)
1x 15ft Rope climb
Rest 3 minutes

Strongman WOD 11
Max rounds in 10 minutes:
3x Axle deadlift (2x bw)
3x Atlas stone ground to shoulder (1.25x bw)
3x Bench press (bw)

Strongman WOD 12
3 rounds:
50ft car push
7x Axle deadlift (1.5x bw)

Strongman WOD 13
For max reps:
Max reps Bench press (bw)
Rest 3 minutes
Max reps Atlas stone over bar (bw)
Rest 3 minutes
Max reps Back squat (bw)
Rest 3 minutes
Max reps Axle deadlift (bw)
Rest 3 minutes
Max reps Atlas stone ground to shoulder (bw)

Strongman WOD 14
5 rounds:
2-4-6-8-10x Atlas stone clean & jerk
4-8-12-16-20x Dynamic stone push-ups

Strongman WOD 15
3 rounds
1 minute max reps Atlas stone (bw) over 52 inch bar
Rest 3 minutes

Strongman WOD 16
5 rounds:
100ft Farmers walk
10x Handstand push-ups

Strongman WOD 17
1RM
Establish a 1RM for 50ft Farmers walk
unlimited time and attempts, rest as needed

Strongman WOD 18
5 rounds
7-5-3-1-1x Atlas stone squats
10x Pull-ups
10x Box jumps (36 inch)
Rest 1 minute

Strongman WOD 19
5 rounds
30x GHD sit-ups
100ft Farmers walk
10x Tire flips
1x 15ft Rope climb
Rest 3 minutes

Strongman WOD 20
3 rounds
15x Keg ground to shoulder
15x Burpees
Rest 2 minutes

Short 'N' Heavy WODs

The following WODs are short duration, metabolic conditioning based workouts utilising Cross Training to build immense strength.

MetCon WOD 1
For time:
25x Thruster
25x Weighted pull-ups
25x Bench press
25x Sumo deadlift high-pull

MetCon WOD 2
4 rounds:
10x each arm KB snatch
15x Wall ball
20x Push-ups

MetCon WOD 3
3 rounds:
10x Power clean (bw)
10x Weight ring dips

MetCon WOD 4
AMRAP in 10 minutes:
5x Deadlift (1.5x bw)
10x Sandbag ground-to-overhead
15x GHD sit-ups

MetCon WOD 5
For time:
Run 400m
50x Pull-ups
50x Push-ups
Run 400m
50x Sit-ups
50x Squats
Run 400m

MetCon WOD 6
5 rounds:
2x Tire flips
3x Back squat
5x Bench press

MetCon WOD 7
AMRAP in 6 minutes
20x Double-unders
5x Deadlifts

MetCon WOD 8
5 rounds:
5-4-3-2-1x Deadlift (1.5x bw)
3x Muscle-up

MetCon WOD 9
9 rounds:
7x Squat clean
8x Burpee box jumps (36 inch)

MetCon WOD 10
AMRAP in 10 minutes:
1 round of Cindy (see 'Girls' benchmark WODs)
3x Clean & jerk

MetCon WOD 11
3 rounds, 21-15-9x reps
Pull-ups
KB swings
Dips

MetCon WOD 12
3 rounds:
1x Deadlift (1RM)
10x Weight pull-ups
25x GHD sit-ups

MetCon WOD 13
8 rounds for max reps:
20 seconds Hang power clean
Rest 10 seconds
20 seconds Push press
Rest 10 seconds

MetCon WOD 14
3 rounds:
30 seconds max reps deadlift
Rest 30 seconds
30 seconds max reps back squat
Rest 30 seconds
30 seconds max reps bench press
Rest 30 seconds

MetCon WOD 15
3 rounds:
7x Deadlift
8x Muscle-ups
9x Squat clean

MetCon WOD 16
5 rounds:
10-8-6-4-2x Back squat
10x Box jump (30 inch)
10x Ring dip

MetCon WOD 17
5 rounds:
10x Deadlift (bw)
10x KB swings
10x Burpee pull-ups

MetCon WOD 18
3 rounds:
1 minute max reps weighted pull-ups
1 minute max reps weighted dips
1 minute rest

MetCon WOD 19
3 rounds:
1 minute max reps Thruster
1 minute max reps weighted pull-ups
1 minute rest

MetCon WOD 20
AMRAP in 8 minutes:
10x Weighted ring dips
Row 250m

One by One WODs

The following WODs utilise a single Cross Training element.

One by One WOD 1
AMRAP:
On the minute every minute perform
1x squat first minute, then rest
2x squats second minute, then rest
3x squats third minute…
Continue until failure

One by One WOD 2
AMRAP:
Perform every minute on the minute, add weight each round until failure
1x Push jerk

One by One WOD 3
5 rounds:
Rest as needed between lifts
Squat clean 1-1-1-1-1x

One by One WOD 4
Time trial:
Row 4km

One by One WOD 5
For time:
Load a sled with 8x 25lb plates
Drag 150 feet, remove a plate, pull/drag back to start
Repeat until down to 1 plate

One by One WOD 6
Max reps in 10 minutes:
Switch arms as necessary, KB may not touch floor
Long cycle KB clean & jerk

One by One WOD 7
Time trial:
Run 10km

One by One WOD 8
Intervals:
Rest 2 minutes between intervals
Row 6x500m

One by One WOD 9
5 rounds:
Rest as needed between rounds
Back squat 5-5-3-3-1x

One by One WOD 10
Intervals:
Row 4x1200m
Rest 2 minutes between intervals

One by One WOD 11
5 rounds for total reps:
45 seconds Box jumps (18 inch)
15 seconds rest
45 seconds Box jumps (24 inch)
15 seconds rest
45 seconds Box jumps (30 inch)
90 seconds rest

One by One WOD 12
AMRAP:
Perform every minute on the minute, add additional weight

each round until failure
2x Front squat

One by One WOD 13
For max rounds:
1x Push jerk
Perform every minute on the minute, add additional weight until failure

One by One WOD 14
Max reps in 12 minutes:
Muscle-ups

One by One WOD 15
For time:
100x Burpee pull-ups

One by One WOD 16
For time:
100x Burpees
On your way to 100 reps you must perform 10 double unders every minute on the minute

One by One WOD 17
For time:
Run 2.7km while holding a 30kg sandbag

One by One WOD 18
1 round:
100x Burpees
On your way to 100 reps you must perform 10x double under every minute on the minute

One by One WOD 19
Rest as needed between lifts:
Thruster 3-3-3-3-3x

One by One WOD 20
For time:
1200m Farmers walk

Minute by Minute WODs

EMOTM WOD 1
Every minute on the minute for 12 minutes:
1x Deadlift
3x Burpees
5x KB swings

EMOTM WOD 2
Every minute on the minute for max rounds:
5x Clapping push ups
15x Kb swings
Each minute thereafter add 1 rep to the push-up, continue until you reach failure

EMOTM WOD 3
Every minute on the minute for max rounds:
1x Thruster
5x Pull-ups
Add 1 rep to thruster each successive minute, continue until you reach failure

EMOTM WOD 4
Every minute on the minute for max rounds:
3x Back squat
5x Strict pull-ups
sprint 40 yards
Each minute thereafter add 1 rep to the squat, continue until you reach failure

EMOTM WOD 5
Every minute on the minute for 12 minutes:
5x Ground to overhead
25x Push-ups

EMOTM WOD 6
Every minute on the minute for 12 minutes:
75ft Farmers walk
After completion rest 5 minutes
75ft yoke carry

EMOTM WOD 7
Every minute on the minute for 8 minutes:
5x Back squats
20x Push-ups

EMOTM WOD 8
Every minute on the minute for 12 minutes:
1x Deadlift
3x Burpees
5x KB swings

EMOTM WOD 9
Every minute on the minute for 15 minutes:
1x Deadlift
1x Hang power clean
1x Front squat
1x Push press

EMOTM WOD 10
Every minute on the minute for 10 minutes:
7x Squat jumps
7x Sprawl
7x Push-ups
7x Sit-ups

EMOTM WOD 11
Every minute on the minute for 12 minutes:
10x Tornado swings
7x/arm KB snatch

EMOTOM WOD 12
Every minute on the minute for 10 minutes:
50ft Farmers walk
3x Ground to shoulder (bw)

EMOTOM WOD 13
Every minute on the minute for 10 minutes:
3x Deadlift (3RM)
10x Ball slams

EMOTOM WOD 14
Every minute on the minute for 12 minutes:
1x Deadlift
3x Burpees
5x KB swings

EMOTOM WOD 15
Every minute on the minute for max rounds:
From the rack start with 1x jerk (50% 1RM)
Add 5 lbs each successive minute, continue until failure

EMOTOM WOD 16
Every minute on the minute for max rounds:
3x Back squat
5x Strict pull-ups
sprint 40 yards
Each minute thereafter add 1 rep to your squat, continue until failure

EMOTOM WOD 17
Every minute on the minute for 15 minutes:
3x Power clean
5x Box jumps (30 inch)
10x Push-ups

EMOTOM WOD 18
Every minute on the minute for max rounds:
5x Box jump (20 inch)
7x Sumo Deadlift high pull
9x Push press

EMOTOM WOD 19
Every minute on the minute for 12 minutes:
75ft Farmers walk
5 minutes recovery
Repeat with 75ft yoke carry

EMOTOM WOD 20
Every minute on the minute for max rounds:
1x Deadlift
Add 25lbs each successive minute, continue until failure.

Bi-Element WODs

The following WODs utilise two different Cross Training elements.

Bi WOD 1
3 rounds:
21-15-9x
Overhead squat
Burpees

Bi WOD 2
5 rounds:
3x Deadlift
15 foot Rope climb, 1x ascent + 20lb vest

Bi WOD 3
AMRAP in 15 minutes:
7x Burpee-pull ups
7x Front squat

Bi WOD 4
AMRAP in 20 minutes:
Add 1 additional rep to each round; 1x-2x-3x-4x etc.
1x Ground to shoulder
1x Muscle-up

Bi WOD 5
10 rounds:
5x KB snatch each arm
10x Thruster

Bi WOD 6
5 rounds:
5x Box jumps (36 inch)
10x 2-arm DB hang muscle snatch

Bi WOD 7
6 rounds:
21x Box jumps (24 inch)
12x Wall-ball

Bi WOD 8
5 rounds:
10x Overhead squat
35x Double-unders

Bi WOD 9
3 rounds:
3x 3 rounds of Cindy (see 'Girls' benchmark section)
40x KB swings

Bi WOD 10
AMRAP in 10 minutes:
10x KB swings
10x Thrusters

Bi WOD 11
5 rounds:
20x Double unders
15 ft Rope climb - 1 ascent

Bi WOD 12
7 rounds:
15x Sumo deadlift high pull
10x Burpees tuck jumps

Bi WOD 13
10 rounds - 10-9-8-7-6-5-4-3-2-1x reps:
Pistols squats
Pull-ups

Bi WOD 14
5 rounds:
6x Snatch
6x Pistol squats

Bi WOD 15
3 rounds:
7x Muscle-ups
21x Thruster

Bi WOD 16
15-12-10x reps:
500m row
DB thrusters
Push-ups
500m row

Bi WOD 17
AMRAP in 7 minutes:
Add 3 additional reps round; 3x-6x-9x-12x etc.
3x Thrusters
3x Pull-ups

Bi WOD 18
5 rounds:
Wall-ball 50-40-30-20-10x
Muscle-ups 10-8-6-4-2x

Bi WOD 19
30 rounds:
2x Pistol squats left leg
2x Pistol squats, right leg
1x Muscle-up

Bi WOD 20
10 rounds:
3x Power snatch
12x Box jumps

Bi WOD 21
3 rounds:
Run 400-800-1200m
Burpees 20-15-10x

Bi WOD 22
7 rounds:
7x Towel pull-ups
7x Ball slams

Bi WOD 23
3 rounds:
21-15-9x
Deadlift
Knees to elbows

Bi WOD 24
AMRAP in 12 minutes
3x Bench press
5x Back squat

Bi WOD 25
5 rounds:
2 minute recovery period between each round
1 minute max reps Front squat
1 minute max reps Box jumps

Tri-Element WODs

The following WODs utilise three different Cross Training elements.

Tri WOD 1
5 rounds:
Squats 80-40-20-40-80x
Push-ups 40-20-10-20-40x
Pull-ups 20-10-5-10-20x

Tri WOD 2
5 rounds:
Row 500-400-300-200-100m
10x Back squats
5x Ring handstand push-ups

Tri WOD 3
AMRAP in 15 minutes:
5x Strict pull-ups
7x Push press
9x Knees to elbows

Tri WOD 4
AMRAP in 12 minutes:
5x L pull-ups
10x Burpees
15x Double unders

Tri WOD 5
10 rounds:
10-9-8-7..3-2-1x reps
Handstand push-ups
Ring dips
Pull-ups

Tri WOD 6
5 rounds:
10x Squat cleans
5x Push-press
3x Overhead squat

Tri WOD 7
AMRAP in 20 minutes:
1x Bear complex
3x Cindy (see 'Girls' benchmark section)
30x Double unders

Tri WOD 8
5 rounds:
1x Power snatch
3x Overhead squat
5x Box jump (24 inch)

Tri WOD 9
3 rounds:
10x Clean & jerk
15x Ring dips
20x KB swings

Tri WOD 10
5 rounds:
30x KB swings
20x DB thrusters
20x Pull-ups

Tri WOD 11
For time:
Row 1000m

25x Deadlifts
50x Burpees

Tri WOD 12
For time:
Run 1000m
30x Handstand push-ups
Row 1000m

Tri WOD 13
AMRAP in 12 minutes:
5x Ground to overhead
10x Floor wipers
15x Lateral hops over BB

Tri WOD 14
6 rounds:
5x Hang power clean
30 yard sprint
Bear crawl back to start

Tri WOD 15
AMRAP in 15 minutes:
3x Thruster
6x Box jump
9x KB swings

Tri WOD 16
For time:
Run 1000m
100x Push-ups
10x Snatch

Tri WOD 17
5 rounds:
8x KB clean & jerk
8x Burpees
8x Strict pull-ups

Tri WOD 18
3 rounds:
1 minute max calorie Row
1 minute max rep Box jump (30 imch)
1 minute max rep KB swing
1 minute rest

Tri WOD 19
3 rounds -21-15-9x reps:
Pull-ups
Push-ups
Squat jumps

Tri WOD 20
AMRAP in 12 minutes:
Row 250m
12x Ball slams
6x Burpees

Tri WOD 21
3 rounds:
10x Standing broad jumps
21x KB swings
24x Push-ups

Tri WOD 22
3 rounds:
Deadlift 9-12-15x
Thruster 15-12-9x
50 yard sprint

Tri WOD 23
11 rounds:
3x Handstand push-ups
7x Knees to elbows
10x Pull-ups

Tri WOD 24
AMRAP in 20 minutes:
10x Pull-ups
5x DB deadlift
8x Push-press

Tri WOD 25
For time:
Row 1000m
25x Deadlifts
50x Burpees

Four or More WODs

The following WODs utilise a minimum of four different Cross Training elements.

Four or More WOD 1
5 rounds:
10x Ring push-ups
20x Sit-ups
30x KB sumo high pulls
40x Squats

Four or More WOD 2
4 rounds:
8x Burpee tuck jumps
8x Knees to elbows
8x Deadlifts
8x Ring dips
8x KB swings
8x Pistols
8x Pull-ups
8x Handstand push-ups

Four or More WOD 3
5 rounds:
5x Muscle-ups
10x Deadlift
15x GHD Sit-ups
Sprint 50 yards

Four or More WOD 4
7 rounds:
7-6-5-4-3-2-1x reps
Clapping push-ups
Squat jumps
Pull-ups
Burpee pull-ups

Four or More WOD 5
3 rounds:
10x Overhead squat
50m Bear crawl
15x KB swings
50m Bear crawl
20x Burpees
50m Bear crawl

Four or More WOD 6
2 rounds:
10x Handstand push-ups
20x Burpees
30x Knees to elbows
40x Push-ups
50x Squats
10x Inverted burpees
20x Pull-ups
30x Box jumps
40x Sit-ups
50x Squat jumps

Four or More WOD 7
3 rounds:
Row 1000m
50x Burpees
50x Box jumps (24 inch)
Run 800m

Four or More WOD 8
2 rounds:
Run 200m
7x Turkish get-up

Run 200m
7x Man-makers
11x Burpee pull-ups

Four or More WOD 9
3 rounds:
20x Double unders
15x Back extensions
10x Ring dips
5x Thrusters

Four or More WOD 10
5 rounds:
5x Muscle-ups
10x Deadlifts
15x GHD sit-ups
Sprint 50 yards

Four or More WOD 11
10 rounds
Run 150m
7x Pull-ups
7x Front squat
7x Handstand push-ups

Four or More WOD 12
5 rounds:
10x Push-ups
20x KB snatch, 10x per arm
30x Sit-ups
40x KB clean, 20x per arm

Four or More WOD 13
4 rounds:
10x Deadlifts
10x Strict pull-up
15x Kettlebell swing
15x Box jump (24 inch)
8x Push press

Four or More WOD 14
6 rounds:
18-15-12-9-6-3x reps
Burpee box jumps (24 inch)
KB swings
Mountain climbers
Sumo deadlift high pull
Wall ball

Four or More WOD 15
5 rounds:
1x Press
1x strict pull-up
1x Squat
3x strict pull-ups
1x Deadlift
5x Strict pull-ups

Four or More WOD 16
3 rounds:
75x wall ball
Run 400m
21x KB swings
12x pull-ups

Four or More WOD 17

3 rounds:
20x KB swings
10x BB push press
15x KB swings
10x BB push press
10x KB swings
15x Push-ups

Four or More WOD 18

5 rounds:
10x KB high pull
10x Sandbag push press
10x Pull-ups
10x Burpees

Four or More WOD 19

AMRAP in 8 minutes:
1x Deadlift
2x Muscle-up
3x Squat clean
4x Handstand push-ups

Four or More WOD 20

3 rounds:
25x Squats
20x Push-ups
26x Lunges
10x Strict pull-ups
50x Flutter kicks
30x Jumping jacks
10x Supermans

Hybrid WODs

The following WODs combine multiple styles of training and exercises along with Cross Training to form a series of hybrid style WODs.

Hybrid WOD 1

5 rounds:
5-4-3-2-1x reps
Thruster
Box jump
Power snatch

Hybrid WOD 2

3 rounds:
20x Double-unders
20x Floor wipers
20x Back extensions
20x MB twists
20x Knees-to-elbows
20x Decline sit-ups

Hybrid WOD 3

3 rounds:
Run 400m
40x Walking lunge steps
30x Sit ups
20x Push ups
10x Burpees

Hybrid WOD 4

3 rounds each:
3x Bench press
10x Plyo push-ups
5x Back squat
6x Box jumps (24 inch)

Hybrid WOD 5
For time:
25x Back squat
50x Box jump (24 inch)
75x Wall ball
100x Squats

Hybrid WOD 6
3 rounds:
15x Burpees
20x Sit-ups
45x Push-ups
60x Squats
Run 400m

Hybrid WOD 7
4 rounds:
20x DB power clean
20x Decline bench abdominal twist
20x Thrusters
20x KB swing
20x Burpees

Hybrid WOD 8
3 rounds – 10 reps per set:
Bench press
KB swings
Overhead squat
Split squats
Thruster

Hybrid WOD 9
5 rounds:
3x Deadlift
5x Thruster
10x Burpees
15x Pull-ups

Hybrid WOD 10
3 rounds:
20x Body row
20x KB swing
20x Squat jumps
20x Push-ups
20x Sit-ups

Hybrid WOD 11
7 rounds:
21-18-15-12-9-6-3x reps
Squat clean
Double unders
Deadlift
Box jump

Hybrid WOD 12
5 rounds:
5x Pull-ups
10x KB swing
5x KB thruster
5x KB Turkish get-up
10x Sledgehammer tire strikes

Hybrid WOD 13
AMRAP in 20 minutes
25x Wall ball
40x sit-ups
5x Ring dips
10x Shuttle run (40m)

Hybrid WOD 14
3 rounds:
Row 500m
30x Box jumps (24 inch)
25x Back extensions
20x Deadlifts

Hybrid WOD 15
3 rounds:
1 minute max reps KB swing
1 minute max reps Thrusters
1 minute max reps Burpee box jumps (24 inch)
1 minute max reps Handstand push-ups
1 minute max reps Wall ball

Hybrid WOD 16
2 rounds:
1000m row
20x Wall ball
30x Push-ups
40x Box jumps
50x Squats
1000m row

Hybrid WOD 17
5 rounds:
4x Dips
12x Pistols
20x Sit-ups
28x KB snatch
Run 50 yards

Hybrid WOD 18
4 rounds
10x Deadlift
10x Wall ball
10x KB swings
10x GHD sit-ups
10x Power clean

Hybrid WOD 19
5 rounds:
12x Deadlifts
20x Pull-ups
12x Clean & jerk
20x Knees to elbows

Hybrid WOD 20
10 rounds:
10x Knees to elbows
10x Ring push-ups
10x L pull-ups

AMRAP WODs

The following WODs are a time trial, designed to see how many rounds of each WOD you can achieve within a set timeframe.

AMRAP WOD 1
AMRAP in 20 minutes:
5x Power cleans
10x Pistol squats
15x Double unders

AMRAP WOD 2
AMRAP in 20 minutes:
15x Squats
10x Push-ups
5x Pull-ups

AMRAP WOD 3
AMRAP in 10 minutes:
5x Clean & jerk
5x Muscle-ups

AMRAP WOD 4
AMRAP in 12 minutes:
6x Bench press
9x Deadlift

AMRAP WOD 5
AMRAP in 20 minutes:
10x Box jumps (24 inch)
10x Pull-ups
20x KB swings
20x Push-ups

AMRAP WOD 6
AMRAP in 20 minutes:
5x Handstand push-ups

10x Pistol squats
15x Deadlifts

AMRAP WOD 7
AMRAP in 10 minutes:
3x Handstand push-ups
6x Sumo deadlift high pulls
4x Thrusters
8x Pull-ups

AMRAP WOD 8
AMRAP in 20 minutes
1x Bear crawl 40m
2x Wall ball
3x Burpees
4x Sit-ups
5x Push-ups
6x Lunges

AMRAP WOD 9
AMRAP in 9 minutes:
3x Deadlift
6x Thruster
Row 200m

AMRAP WOD 10
AMRAP in 20 minutes:
Run 200m
30x KB swings
30x Pull-ups

AMRAP WOD 11
AMRAP in 21 minutes

7x Pull-ups
14x Push-ups
21x Double-unders

AMRAP WOD 12
AMRAP in 8 minutes:
3x Bench press
7x Deadlift

AMRAP WOD 13
AMRAP in 20 minutes:
5x DB thrusters
10x Mountain climbers
15x KB swings

AMRAP WOD 14
AMRAP in 15 minutes:
10x Clean & jerk
20x Deadlift
30x Burpees

AMRAP WOD 15
AMRAP in 10 minutes:
6x Sandbag Turkish get-up
6x KB swing

AMRAP WOD 16
AMRAP in 15 minutes:
1x KB snatch
1x KB overhead squat
1x KB windmill
1x KB jerk
1x KB hand-to-hand swing

AMRAP WOD 17
AMRAP in 20 minutes:
5x Burpee pull-ups
10x Ring dips
15x Sit-ups

AMRAP WOD 18
AMRAP in 10 minutes:
3x Sumo deadlift
7x Ball slams

AMRAP WOD 19
AMRAP in 10 minutes:
3x Power clean
6x Push-ups
9x Knees to elbows

AMRAP WOD 20
AMRAP in 15 minutes:
2x Turkish get-up
10x Zercher squat
12x Lateral hops over bag

AMRAP WOD 21
AMRAP in 20 minutes:
10x Thruster
10x KB swing
10x Burpees

AMRAP WOD 22
AMRAP in 20 minutes:
15x Pull-ups

10x Pistol squats
5x Handstand push-ups

AMRAP WOD 23
AMRAP in 12 minutes:
5x Pull-ups
5x Burpees
5x Ring dips

AMRAP WOD 24
AMRAP in 20 minutes
5x Power cleans
10x Pistol squats
15x Double unders

AMRAP WOD 25
AMRAP in 10 minutes:
3x Deadlift
Row 250m

Epic Endurance Challenges

The following WODs are for the seasoned athlete, designed to test both your physical and mental limits. These workouts aren't pleasant but the feeling of exhilaration upon completion is like no other feeling.

Speed Demon
For time:
Run 3km
Row 3k
Run 1km

Burpee Mile
For time:
Cover a 1600m distance by performing burpees.
Perform a large jump with each rep.

Triple Murph
3 rounds:
1 mile run
100 pullups,
200 pushups,
300 squats
1 mile run
First round to be completed with a weighted vest, partition as necessary
Second round is to be completed without partitions
Third round to be partitioned as necessary

The 500 Challenge
500 pullups
500 pushups
500 situps
500 flutterkicks
500 squats
Partition as necessary

1,500 Rep WOD
10 rounds of:
100 jump ropes
10 burpees
10 situps
10 pushups
10 squats
10 pullups

The Longest Mile
400m of burpees
400m walking lunges
400m bear crawl
400m reverse straight-legged bear crawl

Painstorm XXIV
Run 100m
50 burpees
Run 200m
100 pushups
Run 300m
150 walking lunges
Run 400m
200 squats
Run 300m
150 walking lunges
Run 200m
100 pushups
Run 100m
50 burpees

Frenzy
10 rounds of:
Max burpees 60 seconds

Max pullups 60 seconds
Max tuck jumps 60 seconds
Max jumping jacks 60 seconds
Max distance running 60 seconds

Station 4:00
Station A: running
Station B: burpees
Station C: pullups
Station D: squat jumps
Station E: bear crawl or lunges
Round 1: 5:00 at each station, for total of 25:00.
Round 2: 12:00 at each station, for total of 1:00:00.
Round 3: 30:00 at each station, for total of 2:30:00.
Round 4: 1:00 at each station, for total of 5:00.

Filthy Fifteen Miles
60 rounds of:
Run 400m
3 handstand pushups
2 pistols
1 muscle up

October Breeze
110 minutes: March with rucksack
15 minutes: Eat, hydrate, stretch, change clothes if necessary.
60 minutes: Run at half marathon pace.
60 minutes: Complete 1000 walking lunges.
30 minutes: 5 rounds: ring dips 1:00, rest 1:00, ring pushups 1:00, rest 1:00
60 minutes: Run at half marathon pace.
15 minutes: Eat, hydrate, stretch, change clothes if necessary.
30 minutes: Complete Angie, max intensity.
15 minutes: Sprint 10x100m with 1:00 rests.
15 minutes: Complete 100 burpees.

30 minutes: 4 rounds: 50 squats, 5 muscle ups. Sub 3/3 for MU if necessary.
30 minutes: 500 situps.
10 minutes: Run 1 mile.

Long ladder of doom
Begin with 2 muscle ups, then 4 pistol squats + 2 muscleups, then 6 one-armed pushups + 4 pistol squats + 4 muscle ups, continuing to the rest of the workout at 30.
2 muscle-up
4 pistols
6 one-armed pushups
8 L-pullups
10 toes to bar
12 skin the cats
14 ring dips
16 5 foot broad jumps
18 pushups
20 air squats
22 box jumps
24 lunges
26 double unders
28 burpees
30 jingle-jangles

A Frogman's Christmas
100 dead hang pull-ups
250 push-ups
500 sit-ups
Run 3 miles

Conclusion

I hope you enjoy the plethora of workouts the Cross Training WOD Bible has to offer you, by following these workouts on a regular basis you'll develop not only a strong, flexible, functionally fit body that'll be ready to tackle any situation life throws at it but also an unbreakable mindset and confidence to match.

Whether you're looking to get a competitive advantage in your sport or just to increase your mobility, strength and health these workouts are the answer.

I hope you enjoyed reading this book as much as I enjoyed writing it.

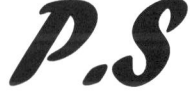

Made in the USA
Lexington, KY
19 March 2016